Amino Acids & Enzymes
What Are They
Why Do You Need Them

Brian B Jacques.

Part of a Series of Mini Health Books
Volume 16

Wisdom For Life Media

Publisher: Wisdom For Life Media

While they have made every effort to verify the information provided in this book, neither the author nor the publisher assumes any responsibility for errors in, omissions from, or different interpretation of the subject matter.

The information herein may be subject to varying laws, regulations, and practices in different areas, states and countries. The purchaser or reader assumes all responsibility for use of the information.

All information included within this book is for educational purposes only. The author and publishers do not attempt to diagnose or treat any medical conditions, be it to do with health, diet or exercise.

If you consider that you have any kind of medical condition, then, you should consult a qualified medical practitioner or doctor before starting any vitamin and/or mineral program or supplement regime, exercise or health training program or diet suggested in this book.

This book is not intended for anyone under the age of 18 years, nor is it intended for breast feeding or pregnant women, underweight people or anyone with eating disorders or a health condition that requires special diets or medical treatment.

The author and publishers disclaim any liability for any loss however caused by anyone using the information contained in this book.

Images

Images are either copyright the author, or are used under the terms of a Royalty Free License.

ISBN - 13: 978-1499666847

ISBN - 10: 1499666845

Contents

Introduction

Amino Acids—The Building Blocks of Proteins

Amino Acids are the building blocks of proteins. They also have a secondary role to play in metabolism.

There are two types of amino acids: essential amino acids which must be obtained from the diet as the body cannot manufacture them itself, and non-essential amino acids which the body can manufacture.

Of the 21 amino acids, 9 of these are essential amino acids. If one of the essential amino acids is missing in the diet, then degradation of body protein's will occur in such areas as muscles, tendons or nails etc..

Essential amino acids are not stored in the body for use later, (unlike fat and starch) and must be included in the diet each day.

Amino acids play a key role in the formation of neurotransmitters as shown in the diagram below, which is also included in the section on enzymes.

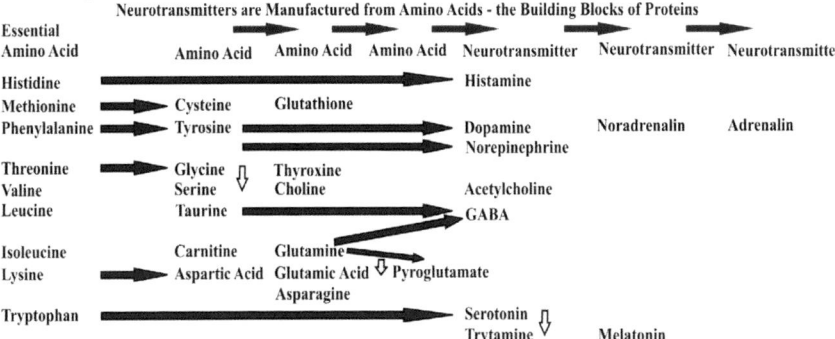

Various proteins make up muscles, tendons, organs, glands, hair, and nails. Proteins not only act as catalysts in the reactions of living cells, but they are also responsible for growth, maintenance and repair of cells too.

Other functions of amino acids include: forming antibodies to combat bacteria and viruses that invade the body, and they form part of the enzyme and hormonal system. Additional activities of amino acids include: building nucleoproteins (RNA and DNA), and carrying oxygen around the body.

Water makes up the largest portion of human bodyweight; the next largest portion is made up of proteins.

Food sources of amino acids include: Meat, poultry, fish, eggs, dairy products, grains, legumes, beans, and nuts. However, if they are lacking in the diet, then the essential ones can be taken as a supplement by capsule or tablet.

Now let us get started with Essential Amino Acids and their function in the human body.

Chapter 1

Essential Amino Acids

Histidine

Histidine is sometimes classed as an essential amino acid. It is found as part of hemoglobin; it has been used for the treatment of rheumatoid arthritis, allergies, ulcers and anemia. It is used for the treatment of digestive ulcers; it is also responsible for the manufacture of red and white blood cells. This amino acid is important for growth and repair of tissues; and is essential for the maintenance of the myelin sheaths which protects nerve cells.

It is a major protector of the body from radiation damage. It assists in lowering blood pressure, and helps in the removal of heavy metals from the body. In addition it facilitates in sexual arousal.

Isoleucine

Helps in the formation of hemoglobin. It is a regulator of blood sugar and a facilitator of energy in the muscle tissues, in addition to being a repair agent for bone, muscle tissue and skin. Isoleucine is often deficient in debilitated individuals.

Leucine

Works with Isoleucine and Valine to promote the healing of muscle tissue breakdown, skin, and broken bones. It acts as a moderator for the uptake of neurotransmitter precursors by the brain to slow the passage of pain signals to the nervous system.

Leucine is recommended for individuals in post-surgery recovery, and for helping to lower blood sugar levels. It acts as an assistant for increasing the production of growth hormones.

Lysine

Ensures an adequate absorption of calcium. It assists in the formation of collagen which forms bones, cartilage and connective tissues. In addition, it helps with the formation of antibodies, hormones and enzymes, which are active fighters against herpes, viral growth and cold sores. It also helps to lower high serum triglyceride levels.

When Lysine is combined with vitamin C, it forms L. Carnitine—a biochemical agent that enables tissue in the muscles to use oxygen more efficiently thus warding off the effects of chronic fatigue.

Methionine

A strong antioxidant and an excellent way to obtain sulfur, that helps prevent problems of the hair, skin pores, and also fingernails. It aids with the breakdown of fats, therefore helping avoid a build-up of fat within the liver and arteries which may prevent the flow of blood to the brain, heart, and kidneys.

Methionine helps to detox harmful agents such as lead along with other heavy metals. It aids in reducing muscle weakness; and helps prevent brittle hair; as well as providing a safeguard against the effects often associated with radiation.

It assists women who take oral birth control pills as it encourages the excretion of estrogen. In addition, it reduces the level of histamine in the body that may cause the brain to relay incorrect communications. Furthermore it is also helpful to individuals experiencing schizophrenia. Methionine is a precursor of cysteine (a sulfur non-essential amino acid) and creatine. It increases levels of glutathione (a powerful antioxidant) and reduces blood cholesterol levels.

Phenylalanine

Manufactures norepinephrine—a neurotransmitter (chemical) that passes messages between nerve cells in the brain. One of its functions is to enhance alertness and wakefulness, as well as boosting memory and reducing pain. Furthermore, it curbs hunger pains and forms a major part of collagen production, in addition to suppressing appetite. It is used to treat arthritis and depression as well as certain motor neuron diseases.

Threonine

Helps in the maintenance of a proper protein balance in the body, in addition to being involved in the formation of collagen, elastin and tooth enamel. It assists in the assimilation of nutrients from food and in metabolism. When it is combined with methionine and aspartic acid (a non-essential amino acid), it blocks the build-up of fats in the liver.

Tryptophan

Tryptophan is especially useful to control hyperactivity in children. As it is a natural relaxant, it helps reduce insomnia by encouraging normal sleep patterns. Tryptophan also eases the effects of anxiety and depression and enhances mood. It acts as an appetite suppressant and is therefore useful in a weight control, program. In addition, it aids in the proper functioning of the immune system and improves the release of growth hormones.

Valine

Valine does a lot of work especially with regard to muscles where it is involved in metabolism, coordination and supplying energy to muscle tissue. It is involved in maintaining a proper nitrogen balance in the body as well as being a treatment for liver and gallbladder disease. It also works in the nervous system where it calms emotions and encourages vigor.

In the next chapter we will look at Non Essential Amino Acids, and the various functions they perform in the human body.

Chapter 2

Non Essential Amino Acids

Alanine

This non-essential amino acid is needed if a person does aerobic exercise as it guards against a toxic build-up in muscle cells which is generated when exercising and more energy is expended by the body. Alanine also plays a role in glucose metabolism that the body converts to energy.

Arginine

Often used in an erectile dysfunction program, arginine increases blood flow to the penis, in addition to increasing sperm count; it is very important for proper functioning of the immune system, especially in retardation of tumor growth and cancer proliferation. It stimulates the thymus gland to make T cells—a vital constituent of the immune system. In addition, it promotes the release of insulin from the pancreas, as well as reducing alcohol toxicity and neutralizing ammonia.

In a weight loss program it is important for reducing body fat and increasing muscle mass. It assists in the discharge of growth hormones to facilitate muscle growth and tissue repair.

Arginine is an important constituent of collagen which makes it especially useful for arthritic conditions and inflamed tissue disorders.

Aspartic Acid

Is involved in the function of RNA and DNA which are transporters of genetic information such as identity. It also acts as a carrier of specific minerals through the small intestine into the bloodstream for use by body cells. Aspartic Acid is intimately involved in revitalizing cell formation and activity, as well as being involved in metabolism.

It merges with other amino acids to create molecules that absorb and remove toxins from the bloodstream. In addition, it also purges ammonia from the liver.

As it is also involved in increasing stamina, it is excellent for those suffering from chronic fatigue and depression.

Cysteine

I have always had an interest in the actions of sulfur compounds in the body, and here we have cysteine (or to give it its full name, N-acetyl cysteine (NAC)—a sulfur non-essential amino acid—that is linked to the essential (sulfur) amino acid methionine. Another sulfur amino acid homocysteine is also involved here too.

Cysteine has important functions to perform, including: acting as a powerful antioxidant and protector of the liver and brain from the effects of alcohol, drugs and smoking.

Cysteine also helps prevent hardening of the arteries and eases the pain of rheumatoid arthritis. Additionally, it helps burn fat and builds muscle, as well as facilitating recovery from burns.

Homocysteine

Homocysteine can be a harmful amino acid. It is not obtained from the diet. Instead, it is synthesized from methionine by the addition of adenosine triphosphate (ATP). ATP is responsible for transporting chemical energy within cells for metabolism. The addition of ATP creates a catalytic action to form S-adenosylmethionine (SAMe). This is an intermediate process which ultimately forms homocysteine.

Homocysteine has two main roles: It can be converted back to methionine with the aid of vitamin B12 (cyanocobalamin) or used to create cysteine and alpha-ketobuterate with the aid of vitamin B6 (pyridoxine) and vitamin B9 (folic acid).

If B vitamins are lacking in the body, then the conversion of homocysteine back to methionine or to cysteine can be greatly reduced. If this happens, then homocysteine can form a sticky plaque on arterial walls. For this reason, it is linked to an increased risk of heart disease, stroke and dementia. Additionally homocysteine levels rise with age and if a person smokes.

Glutamic Acid

Glutamic Acid acts as a fuel for the brain by increasing mental capacity in addition to being an excitatory neurotransmitter for the nervous system and spinal cord. It is important for sugar and fat metabolism, and is a carrier of potassium into the spinal fluid. It helps correct personality disorders and is a precursor of arginine, glutamine, glutathione (a very potent antioxidant), ornithine, proline, and gamma-amino-butyric acid (GABA)—a neurotransmitter that is synthesized in the brain.

Glutamine

The most abundant amino acid which plays a critical role in immune system performance. It is used along with Omega-3 essential fatty acids to treat a leaky gut. It has an important role to play in building and maintaining muscle tissue. Additionally, it helps prevent muscle wasting that can be the result of extended bed rest or such diseases as AIDS and cancer.

Glutamine is important for maintaining the pH (acid/alkaline balance) of the body as well as assisting in maintaining digestive and intestinal system health.

It is also considered a "brain food" as it assists in memory function and concentration, as well as providing a source of energy. In addition, it relieves instances of impotence and fatigue.

Glycine

Especially useful to calm aggressive and manic depressive individuals. It is involved in supporting a healthy nervous system and assists in making several other amino acids. It is an integral part of hemoglobin and cytochromes—enzymes which are involved in energy production. Glycine is involved in the manufacture of glucagon which activates glycogen for energy.

Ornithine

Assists in stimulating the release of growth hormones which encourages the metabolism of body fat. This effect is increased with the addition of arginine and carnitine.

Ornithine is an important component of a strong immune system as well as being involved in purging ammonia, and liver regeneration.

It facilitates insulin secretion and assists insulin's vocation as a muscle building hormone.

Proline

Partners with vitamin C to elevate healthy connective tissue. It enhances skin texture by assisting with the production of collagen. Proline plays a role in cartilage healing and reinforcement of joints, tendons and the heart muscle.

Serine

Serine is a part of the myelin sheaths that cover and protect nerve fibers. It is a component in DNA and RNA function (which are transporters of genetic information such as identity), as well as cell formation.

It supports the immune system by producing immunoglobulins and antibodies to fight infections. In addition, it helps metabolise fats and fatty acids as well as being a storage source of glucose by the liver and muscles.

Taurine

Taurine is critical for the proper use of calcium, magnesium, potassium and sodium. It is a key component of good vision by helping prevent macular degeneration. It is also an important component of bile which is required by the digestive system to break down fats.

Taurine aids in the cleansing of free radical waste and helps control many aspects of the aging process within the body. It is important for circulatory system health for those people who suffer from atherosclerosis, cardiac arrhythmias or hypertension (high blood pressure).

Taurine provides neurotransmitter activity in areas of the brain and retina.

Tyrosine

Tyrosine is important for the correct functioning of the glandular and nervous systems. As a regulator of mood and depressive tendencies, tyrosine is a precursor of adrenaline, norepinephrine and dopamine, and works with the thyroid, adrenal and pituitary glands to fulfil this role.

It contains melanin which is the pigment responsible for hair and skin color.

It also assists in cases of chronic fatigue and low sex drive, allergies and headaches.

Chapter 3

Enzymes

All living things contain enzymes. Enzymes basically are large biological molecules that perform many thousands of chemical conversions in the body that are essential for life. They are involved in everything from the digestion of food to the synthesis of DNA. The majority of enzymes are proteins, and some may use a co-factor such as biotin (one of the B vitamins), magnesium or iron to carry out their function.

In an enzyme reaction, molecules at the beginning of the process called substrates are converted through the actions of the enzyme into other molecules called products.

The performance of enzymes can be affected by such things as the pH of the body, body temperature, and inhibitors. Some drugs contain inhibitors to interfere with the performance of an enzyme. An example of inhibitors is medications used to delay the metabolic enzyme acetylcholinesterase from breaking down a brain neurotransmitter acetylcholine to help improve memory function.

Enzymes are not just confined to functions of the body. Some enzymes are used in commercial applications such as in biological washing powder where enzymes are used to remove fat stains from clothes. Enzymes are a component of meat tenderizers which break down proteins in the meat which makes it easier to chew.

In this book I am not concerned with the commercial application of enzymes, but in what functions they perform in the body.

Enzymes work as catalysts to produce energy. Enzymes are capable of performing these tasks because, unlike food proteins such as casein in egg albumin, gelatin, or soy protein, they are catalysts. This means that by their mere presence, and without being consumed in the process, enzymes can speed up chemical processes that would otherwise run very slowly, if at all. So in a nutshell, unlike vitamins and minerals, which are the building blocks of various body functions, enzymes are the body's workers—they make things happen. But very few people know about the vital role that enzymes play in maintaining a healthy body.

There are 3 broad classifications of enzymes

A) Those that occur naturally in our food

B) Those that are made in the body from digestion of food (approximately 24 in total)

C) Metabolic enzymes made to run the biochemical reactions occurring in the body

I have provided a list of some of these enzymes and what body function they perform later in this book.

Each enzyme is designed to do a specific job that no other enzyme can fulfill. A protease enzyme (which breaks down protein) will not break down carbohydrates; likewise an enzyme whose job it is to break down milk sugar and milk protein (a job for lactase) will not break down fats (that is a job for lipase).

Therefore, the chemical shape of each enzyme is specialized so that it can initiate a reaction only in certain substances (called substrates), or a group of closely related chemical substrates, and not in others.

It can be best described as having a lock and key effect. The substrate must have the correct "key" profile in order to enter the enzyme lock. If it doesn't then it will be rejected and then will have to look elsewhere for the correct enzyme. After performing a function, an enzyme does not degrade. In other words, it can be reused many times. This "making and breaking" process happens many times each second.

I have included a diagram at the end of this chapter so you can see how this enzyme actions works.

To give you an idea of how many different enzymes are involved in various body processes, take the breakdown of glucose to carbon dioxide and water. This action requires 19 different chemical reactions which involves 19 specific enzymes.

Nature planned for food enzymes to play an important role in the digestion of our food. Scientists say that digestive problems are a major health hazard in modern society. To explain the importance of enzymes is not easy, but my goal is to present an understanding of the role that enzymes play in keeping you healthy.

All raw, uncooked fruit, vegetables, meat, and poultry contain enzymes that play a necessary role in virtually all of the biochemical activations that bring our foods to maturity or ripeness. And when the conditions are right (the enzymes have not been killed off by food processing or over-cooking), they will assist in the digestion of the food in which they are contained. If food enzymes do some of the work, the body is not burdened with eliminating an accumulation of food it cannot assimilate.

To give you an example of enzymes at work, think of an apple. An apple is a very complex structure containing various starches, sugars, fiber, malic acid and enzymes, and the skin of the apple provides a protective coat.

A chain-reaction starts as soon as you cut into the skin of an apple. And you can see the result of this chain-reaction within 15 minutes as the white inner part starts to turn brown. This is the action of enzymes on the sugars and starches which has started a decaying and fermenting process within the apple structure.

I have included a list on the next page of some of the foods that contain digestive enzymes and what they do.

	Amylase (Digests Sugars)	Protease (Digests Protein)	Lipase (Digests Fat)	Peroxidase & Catalase (Disarms Free Radicals)
Apples				*
Bananas	*			
Cabbage	*			
Eggs (Uncooked)	*	*	*	*
Grapes				*
Honey (Raw/unpasturised)	*			*
Kidney Beans	*	*		*
Mangoes				*
Milk (Raw/Unpasturised)	*			*
Mushrooms	*	*		*
Pineapple	*	*		
Rice	*			
Soy Beans		*		
Sweet Corn	*			*
Sweet Potatoes		*		
Wheat	*	*		

Food allergies, gas and bloating, heartburn, and constipation or diarrhea are problems that can result from a lack of enzymes. Studies are gradually revealing that the resulting metabolic problems may be the direct cause of many chronic degenerative diseases.

To ensure that you get adequate enzymes, it is preferable to take enzyme supplements. These usually come in either enteric coated capsules (enteric meaning it will dissolve in the stomach or small intestine, and not before it gets to where it is supposed to work) or in tablet form.

Full spectrum enzyme supplements are available which means they contain enzymes that will assist in the breakdown of protein, carbohydrates, fats and starches. You may also see "proteolytic enzymes". These are in fact protease enzymes that break down proteins into their smallest elements (peptides). There is a large selection of enzyme supplements available. Make sure you purchase one that is manufactured by a reputable supplier.

Sometimes an enzyme formula will contain hydrochloric acid (a stomach acid), which helps in the breakdown of foods in the stomach. As a person ages, the body produces less of this acid, which can result in digestive problems and malabsorption of nutrients. If you have eaten a meal and feel as if you have a heavy weight in your stomach, then you may be lacking hydrochloric acid.

Here is a diagram to show you how enzymes work. Notice the sucrose substrate and its keyway, and the sucrase enzyme with the correct "lock" to receive it. In this illustration a sucrose substrate is converted into fructose and glucose (called a "product") by the action of the sucrase enzyme. These products will go on to perform other body functions.

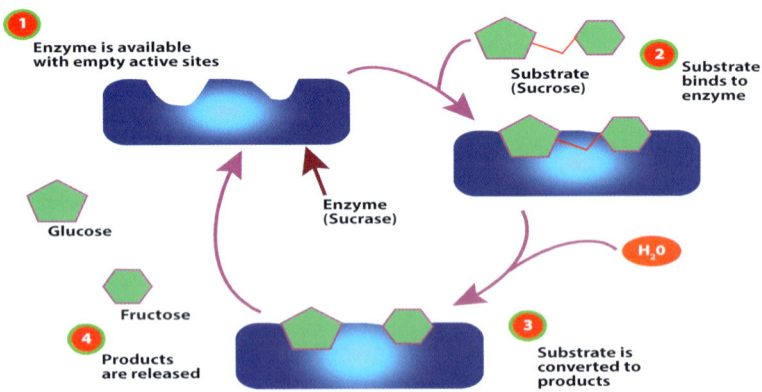

Chapter 4

Enzymes and Minerals

Minerals are the spark plugs of life because they are required to act as co-factors in the activation of thousands of enzyme reactions within the body.

They are more important than vitamins since plants manufacture vitamins within their own structure, but minerals must be obtained from the soil.

Magnesium

Works with Vitamin B1 and B6 to assist in correct enzyme function—especially protein synthesis.

Zinc

Is needed to make stomach acid and protein splitting enzymes—proteases.

Iron

Is needed for enzymes involved in energy metabolism.

Copper

Works with enzymes involved in iron metabolism.

Molybdenum

Is a constituent of various enzymes.

Calcium

Works with enzymes involved in nerve transmissions.

Minerals also help to regulate the pH (acid alkaline balance) of the body.

Chapter 5

pH Balance Body Temperate and Enzymes

The pH balance of the body, the body temperature and the effectiveness of enzymes are all inter-related. Each enzyme operates at its own optimum pH level, as well as its optimum body temperature level.

It is probably easier to explain if you view the following diagrams.

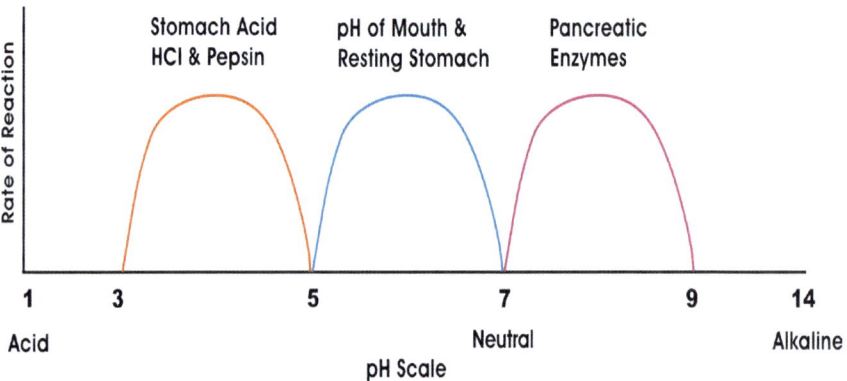

Let me start with the pH scale. You can determine your body's pH by using testing papers which are obtainable from drugstores. You need to use two test strips. Put a small amount of saliva on one and a small sample of urine on the other. Do not use the same test strip for both samples. Along with the test strips, there should be a color scale. Now compare your test strips with the color scale, to ascertain if your body is acidic or alkaline. A balanced pH is a figure of 7 on the scale.

The majority of people who live in the United States as well as Western Europe are acidic. This has much to do with the type of food that is eaten. As a high proportion of the diet is from a high fat source such as red meat and/or processed foods which can contain a high proportion of sodium, sugar, preservatives and artificial colors, in addition to a lack of fiber and exercise. This tends to make the body acidic—a condition known as acidosis. Acidosis can lead to inflammation in the body which can develop into such conditions as osteoarthritis, hypertension (high blood pressure), heart disease, stroke and diabetes.

It is relatively easy to bring the body back into a balanced state. Minerals are very alkalizing, especially calcium and magnesium supplements, chlorophyll in liquid form (chlorophyll is derived from alfalfa), and by eating alkalizing foods such as tomatoes, and the majority of fruits and vegetables. This is by no means a complete list. Note. While most citrus fruits are acidic, when they have been digested they are alkaline forming.

Acidic foods to avoid would be mainly beef, pork, lamb, butter and peanut butter to name a few. There are some excellent acid/alkaline food lists available on the Internet. Just type "acid alkaline food lists" into your search engine.

After you have been alkalizing your body for one month, use two test strips to do the saliva and urine test again to see if your body has become more alkaline. If you are now in the balanced zone, you have made good corrections to your diet, and this is the diet to follow in future. If your body is still acidic, then you have a bit more work to do.

One thing to bear in mind. The majority of degenerative diseases are caused by an acidic environment which causes inflammation. In addition, instances of cancer and the proliferation of cancer cells are more common in an acidic body. And finally, parasite and worm infestations thrive in an acidic body, as does candida yeast.

Let us now turn to body temperature, as this has a direct bearing on the effectiveness of enzyme use and production.

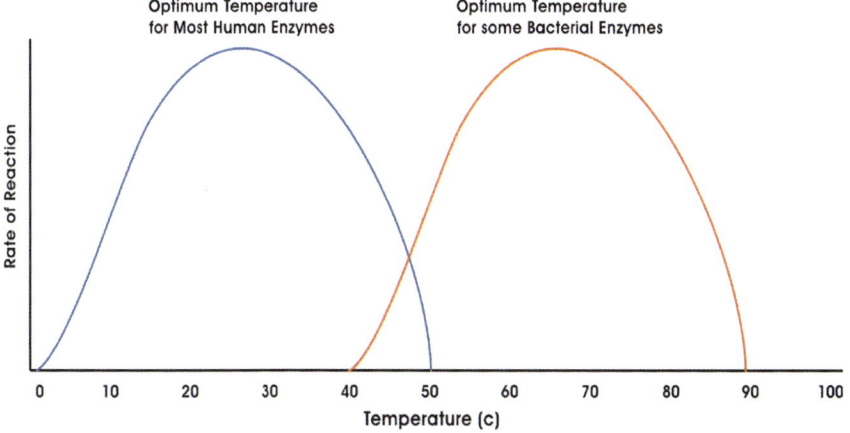

If you look at the temperature graph you can see the optimum temperature for human enzymes is around 25–30 degrees Celsius (77—86 degrees Fahrenheit). Below this they will be rather sluggish to get going, and above this at 50 degrees Celsius (122 degrees Fahrenheit) they will degrade.

Bacterial enzymes which work in the intestines operate at a higher temperature, the optimum being around 65—70 degrees Celsius (149—158 degrees Fahrenheit). Below this they will not be as effective, and above this they will degrade.

So what affects body temperature? All manner of different things. If you are out in extremely cold weather, then your body temperature can drop quite dramatically. If this occurs for a lengthy period of time, then it can affect the effectiveness of enzymes in your body.

Likewise, if your body gets too hot—if you are in a very hot climate for example, or if you have a fever and run a high temperature, then this can have an impact on the enzymes in your body.

One thing to remember. Your body is a very delicate machine, and it will take a lot of abuse before it lets you know that something is wrong. But heed what it is telling you, and look after it. After all, it is the only one that you have.

Chapter 6

You Have Something To Eat—What Happens Next

I'm Hungry! So you have something to eat. So, what happens next?

Mouth

When food is chewed, saliva containing amylase enzymes starts to work on digesting carbohydrates. These enzymes together with your chewing action start the breakdown of the food. You swallow the food; it then passes down the esophagus into the stomach.

Amylase enzymes stop working in the stomach as it is too acidic for them.

Stomach

Protein is not digested in the mouth but in the stomach where the addition of hydrochloric acid (HCI) does the work.

Protein is broken down into smaller collections of amino acids called Peptides. This is done by the activation of a protein digesting enzyme called pepsin.

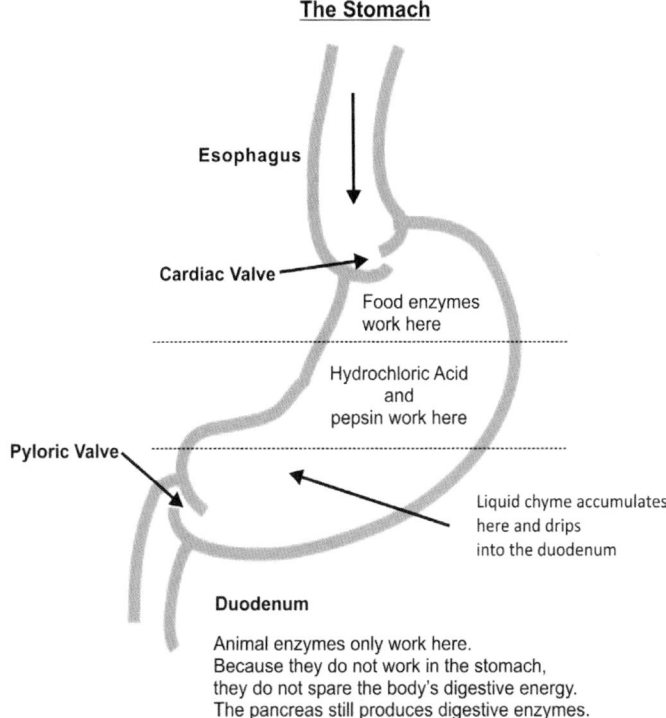

The Stomach

Esophagus

Cardiac Valve

Food enzymes work here

Hydrochloric Acid and pepsin work here

Pyloric Valve

Liquid chyme accumulates here and drips into the duodenum

Duodenum

Animal enzymes only work here.
Because they do not work in the stomach, they do not spare the body's digestive energy. The pancreas still produces digestive enzymes.

Liver

A green liquid called Bile is made in the Liver and stored in the gall bladder. Bile contains lecithin which helps break down fats.

Pancreas

Once Peptides leave the stomach they meet peptidase enzymes from the pancreas. This breaks them down into individual amino acids ready for absorption.

The pancreas produces enzymes to break down carbohydrates, fats and proteins. In addition, vitamin B6 is needed for this process.

Duodenum

Protein digestion continues in the first part of the small intestine called the duodenum This is done by the secretion of digestive enzymes produced in the pancreas and liver.

Because this is a more alkaline environment, amylase enzymes secreted from the pancreas continue the digestion of carbohydrates.

Small Intestine

Amylase enzymes secreted from the small intestine and the pancreas complete the work of breaking down carbohydrates.

Food particles are mixed with bile and enzymes from the pancreas and peptidase from the small intestine.

Large Intestine

Indigestible food plus water are processed, stored and disposed of.

Rectum

Solid waste passes from the rectum to the anus so it can be evacuated from the body.

Chapter 7

How Are The Brain And Gut Connected?

Many people are under the impression that all thought processes are done by the brain, but this is not so. The digestive system plays a large role as well. Did you know that the gastrointestinal tract (or gut for short) produces two thirds of the body's serotonin—the neurotransmitter that puts you in a good mood; and that the overall digestive system produces over 100 million neurons and as many neurotransmitters as the brain itself.

So consider this! Every time you eat a meal signals go to the brain, because the brain and digestive system are in permanent contact with each other. This may explain to you why certain foods will give you a good feeling, while other types of food will make you irritable or depressed. Therefore consuming good nutrition is not just about eating, it is about being able to digest the food and absorb it as well. And digestive enzymes play a critical role in this process.

Chapter 8

Digestive Enzymes and Their Function

Here is a list of some of the digestive enzymes and the function they perform.

Alpha Chymotrypsin
Is activated by Trypsin in the small intestine to assist in the breakdown of protein.

Alpha Galactosidase
Aids in the breakdown of complex carbohydrates commonly found in fruits and vegetables that are difficult to digest.

Amylase (Mycozyme)
Digests starches.

Betaine (HCI)
Assists in the breakdown of fats and proteins. Helps in increasing hydrochloric acid in the stomach.

Bromelain
From pineapple. A proteolytic enzyme which assists in the breakdown of protein. It also has anti-inflammatory properties, and is effective over a broad pH range.

Bile Salts
Emulsify fats and prepare them for further digestion by the enzyme Lipase.

Cellulase
Helps breakdown the cellular structure of plant fibres.

Glucoamylase
Digests glucose sugars.

Invertase
Aids in the breakdown of sucrose (sugar) into glucose and fructose.

Lactase
Aids in the breakdown of milk sugar and milk protein.

Lipase
Assists in the breakdown of dietary fats.

Malt Diastase
Transforms starch into maltose and then into glucose.

Pancreatin
Is produced by the pancreas to digest proteins, carbohydrates, and fats in the small intestine.

Papain
Digests proteins.

Pectinase
Breaks down pectin in fruit.

Pepsin
Is used for the digestion of proteins.

Peptidase
Aids in the breakdown of proteins.

Phytase
Assists in breaking down legumes, corn, seeds and grains. Assists in breaking down phytic acid in oil seeds and grains which cannot be digested by the body.

Protease
Aids in the breakdown of proteins.

Rennin
Assists in the breakdown of milk proteins in the stomach.

Serrapeptase
A proteolytic enzyme that assist in the breakdown of non-living tissue, also helps reduce inflammation and arterial plaque.

Trypsin
Produced within the pancreas and is secreted into the small intestine where it helps regulate other enzymes and assists in breaking down arginine residue and lysine. Trypsin converts peptides (small protein molecules) into amino acids which assists in the absorption of protein from food.

Chapter 9

To Sum Up What Digestive Enzymes Do

- Enzymes turn food into fuel for each body cell:
    - Muscle cells
    - Brain cells
    - Immune cells
    - Blood cells
- They also make the heart beat and they are also involved in nerve transmissions.
- Vitamins and minerals are needed to make enzymes work.
- Enzymes prepare food for absorption.
- Protein is broken down into amino acids.
- Complex Carbohydrates are broken down into simple sugars.
- Fats are broken down into fatty acids and glycerol.
- Each day 2 gallons of digestive juices produced by the pancreas, liver, stomach and small intestine pour into the digestive tract.
- The body needs an adequate supply of nutrients to make digestive enzymes.

Chapter 10

Metabolic Enzymes

Metabolic enzymes need good nutrients and the digestive enzymes to provide the fuel that they need to perform their various functions. Some metabolic enzymes need minerals—especially magnesium and zinc to act as co-factors for their synthesis and the actions they perform in the body. It is very difficult to describe all that they do, and how many of them that there are—there are literally hundreds of them—each performing their own particular function in the body.

One thing to bear in mind with metabolic enzymes—you do not get them from supplements—the body has to have the necessary nutrients to be able to produce them itself.

Some of the vital functions they are involved in include:

• The Nervous System

• Motor Function

• Memory

• Neurotransmitters

The pancreas is a vital organ for the production of metabolic enzymes. These enzymes have the ability to act as catalysts for various chemical reactions within body cells. These reactions include energy production, detoxification, blood purification, and the processing of nutrients from digested food. This processing action turns these nutrients into various cells required for the production of muscles, nerves, bones, blood, and lung cells. In addition, these enzymes also help to purify the blood.

Chapter 11

The Importance of Neurotransmitters and the Lecithin Connection

I have mentioned neurotransmitters, but what are they and what do they do? Neurotransmitters are manufactured from amino acids— the building blocks of protein. The metabolic enzymes role here is to breakdown the neurotransmitter so that an excess does not form. In other words, the neurotransmitter and metabolic enzyme work in harmony with each other.

To help with our discussion, take a look at the diagram below. The gap between the transmitting neuron and the receiving neuron is called the synapse. Current studies estimate that the average male human brain contains 86 billion neurons.

There are many synapses around each neuron, and they come in different shapes to accommodate the shape of the neuron. Synapses are very tiny at approximately 20-40 nanometers (nm) wide. For an idea of scale, one inch is about 25.4 million nm long. The thickness of a single sheet of paper is about 100,000 nm. I had to create the diagram with a very wide synapse in order to demonstrate the function of the neurotransmitter and metabolic enzyme.

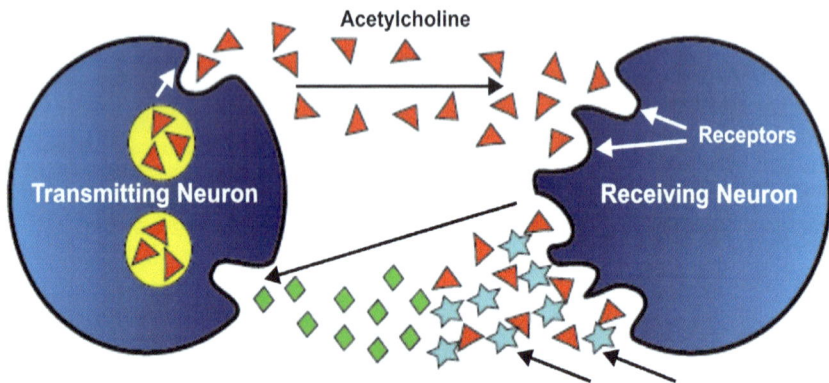

After signaling, acetylcholine is released from receptors and broken down by the metabolic enzyme acetylcholinesterase. The acetylcholine will then be recycled in a continuous process

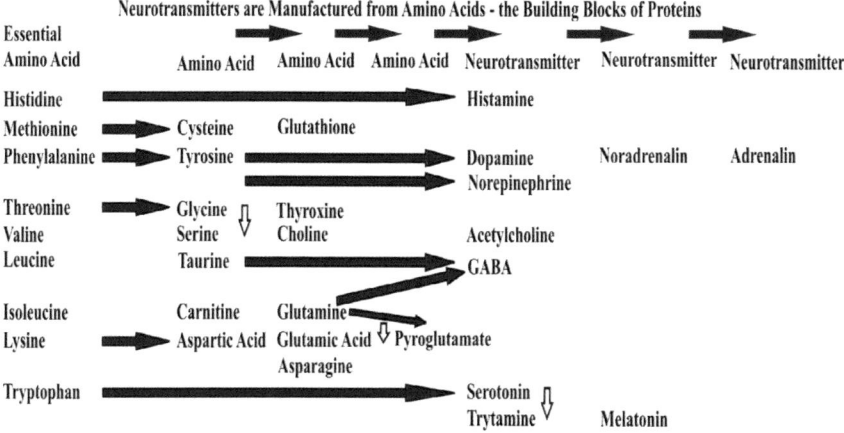

Neurotransmitters are Manufactured from Amino Acids - the Building Blocks of Proteins

Acetylcholine the memory neurotransmitter is formed from amino acids as demonstrated in the diagram above. It is a critical component of memory retention, and is not as one might think—an electronic component that you might find in a radio for example, but are in fact chemicals found in the brain that are responsible for the transmission of signals between neurons across the space between nerve cells (neurons), or as it is sometimes called the synapses. Neurotransmitters stimulate muscle fibers to contract or neurons to send a chemical message to other neurons.

I am sure that you have heard of Alzheimer's disease. Scientists have discovered that Alzheimer's disease is linked to low levels of acetylcholine (part of the cholinergic system) in the hippocampus and neocortex regions of the brain.

Whilst acetylcholine is known as the "memory" neurotransmitter, in fact other neurotransmitters are involved as well. You may have heard of one of these—serotonin which is linked to being in a good mood. These other neurotransmitters have specific functions to perform within the nervous system and for memory function.

Metabolic enzymes are also implicated in memory retention as well. One of these, acetylcholinesterase has the function to break down acetylcholine. But what if there is insufficient acetylcholinesterase to break down the acetylcholine? Well, an individual can become hyperactive as a result. It is important to remember that this forming of the neurotransmitter and the metabolic enzyme breaking it down happens many times each second—as shown in the diagram, it is a continuous process.

Superoxide Dismutase (SOD) is another example of a metabolic enzyme. It has antioxidant properties which assist in the neutralizing of the free radical superoxide. All free radicals can be highly destructive to body cells, and especially if they attack the major organs of the body. I have described free radicals and antioxidants in the next chapter.

So where does lecithin come into the equation? The word lecithin comes from the Greek word Lekithos meaning egg-yolk. It was first discovered in 1805 by French scientist Maurice Gobley when he separated a fat-like substance from egg-yolk.

Egg-yolk was the prime source of lecithin until the 1930's when it was discovered that soy-lecithin could be extracted from the waste by-products of soy bean production. Today, the majority of lecithin is now derived from soy, although it can be obtained from wheat germ, peanuts, cauliflower, cabbage, grape juice and liver as well.

Lecithin is not classed as an essential fatty acid as it can be produced in the liver as well as obtained from the diet. Essential fatty acids like essential amino acids are not made in the body, but must be obtained from the diet.

Lecithin is one of the best sources of phospholipids—important mood enhancers as well as being intimately involved in protecting you against memory decline as you get older. There are several different phospholipids, but the two most important ones are Phosphatidyl Choline and Phosphatidyl Serine. The neurotransmitter acetylcholine is built from choline derived from Phosphatidyl Choline. In addition, acetylcholine is an important component of the myelin sheaths which layers brain cells and the spinal cord to protect it from damage. It also accelerates messages passed between various nerve cells.

Phosphatidyl Choline is made up of B vitamins, phosphoric acid, choline, gamma linoleic acid and inositol. In addition to its function in helping build acetylcholine; it is also one of the key building blocks of cell membranes in addition to being a protector against cell oxidation. It is one of only two nutrients needed by the liver to break down fats. The other is methionine— an essential amino acid, derived from protein. The liver expels fats which are turned into energy for use by the body.

Lecithin is transported throughout the circulatory and nervous systems and, in conjunction with different metabolic enzymes, performs many important functions in the body in addition to those described above. It is an excellent emulsifier in helping lower blood cholesterol; in helping correct liver and nervous system disorders and in combating atherosclerosis, which if left unchecked can lead to a heart attack or stroke. Many people also take it as part of a weight loss program.

Lecithin is not only used for good health. It is also used in the manufacturer of paints, textiles, lubricants and waxes; in food processing, chocolate, butter and margarine manufacture, and in the cosmetics industry.

Superoxide Dismutase (SOD) is another example of a metabolic enzyme. It has antioxidant properties which assist in the neutralizing of the free radical superoxide. All free radicals can be highly destructive to body cells, and especially if they attack the major organs of the body.

Chapter 12

Understanding Free Radicals and Antioxidants

What are free radicals? Why do they damage the human body? How is it that vitamins A (and its precursor beta carotene), E and C can help protect the body from free radical damage? It is important to understand why eating at least five serving each day of antioxidant rich fruits and vegetables, along with suitable antioxidant supplements will benefit your health, and help prevent cancer, heart disease, memory loss and other illnesses from developing.

To start, let us look at free radicals. Where do they come from, and what damage do they do. Everyone has free radicals—they are part of living. They come from the metabolism of the food you eat as well as from environmental factors such as air pollution, radiation, cigarette smoke, herbicides, household cleaners, skin care products, cosmetics—in fact anything that has a chemical element in it. Even the immune system can develop free radicals to help destroy bacteria and viruses.

Free radicals are atoms or groups of atoms with an odd or un-impaired number of electrons. These can be formed when oxygen interacts with certain molecules.

These highly reactive molecules can start a chain reaction—like a falling pack of cards. The danger is the damage they can do when they come into contact with important cellular components such as DNA or cell membranes. Cells can die if this occurs.

Some of the degenerative conditions caused by free radicals:
- Deterioration of the eye lens, which contributes to cataracts or blindness.
- Inflammation of the joints (arthritis).
- Damage to nerve cells in the brain, which can result in Parkinson's or Alzheimer's disease.
- Acceleration of the aging process.
- Increased risk of coronary heart disease since free radicals encourage low-density lipoprotein (LDL) cholesterol to adhere to artery walls in the form of arterial plaque.
- Certain cancers triggered by damaged cell DNA.

This is where antioxidants come in. The main antioxidant vitamins are vitamin A (and its precursor beta carotene), vitamin C and vitamin E. There are also antioxidant minerals such as selenium and zinc, and antioxidant herbs such as ginkgo biloba and garlic which support the circulatory system, and turmeric which supports memory function.

Antioxidants neutralize free radicals by donating one of their own electrons thus ending the electron stealing cycle. The antioxidants don't become free radicals themselves as they have spare electrons and are stable in either form. They act as protectors and help to prevent tissue and cell damage which could lead to disease.

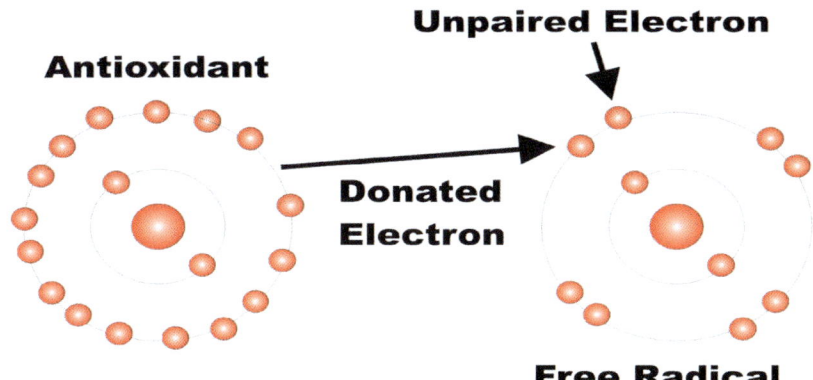

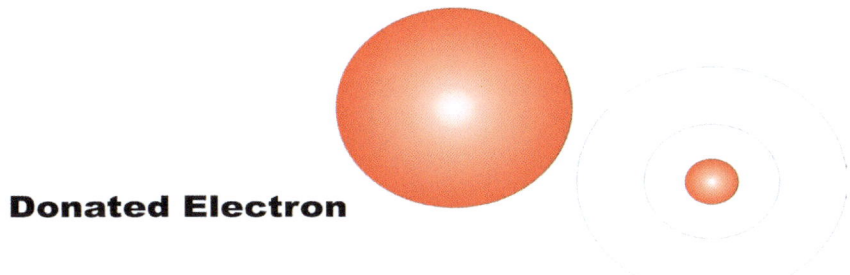

Chapter 13

Antioxidants and Disease Prevention

The greatest killers in the Western world are heart disease, stroke and cancer. Vitamin E is the most abundant fat soluble antioxidant in the body. It is one of the main defenders against oxidation and helps protect you against cardiovascular disease by helping to neutralize the effects of LDL (low density lipoprotein)–the "bad" cholesterol and plaque formation which blocks arteries and can lead to a heart attack and stroke.

The most abundant water soluble antioxidant is vitamin C. Vitamin C helps to neutralize free radical formations caused by cigarette smoke and other forms of air pollution. Also many studies have shown that high doses of vitamin C equate to lower rates of cancer especially of the mouth, larynx and esophagus.

Antioxidants are the best vitamins and minerals for boosting your memory. In addition to vitamins A (and its precursor beta carotene), C and E already mentioned, we can also add the minerals zinc and selenium, as well as co-enzyme Q10 and the herbs ginkgo biloba and turmeric all of which have antioxidant properties too. Antioxidants supply essential oxygen to the brain as well as helping prevent the process of oxidation.

Elevated antioxidant levels equate to a clearer mind. Researchers in Switzerland and the US have found that people with the highest scores in memory tests have elevated levels of vitamin E, vitamin C and vitamin A.

Researchers speculate that one of the reasons for this is that antioxidants have a beneficial effect on the circulatory system by reducing artery disease and improving circulation to the brain.

Inflammation is linked to many diseases in the body, from arthritis to cardiovascular disease, and it appears that as arteries become damaged, so does the brain. Antioxidants play a key role in reducing inflammation and in preventing oxidation in the brain.

Inflammation often equates to pain, redness or swelling—especially in the joints— which is the body's way of telling you that something is amiss. Therefore it seems that reducing inflammation is one of the keys to restoring your body's health, and this is where antioxidants play a crucial role. Each of the body's systems is interlinked. And something that may seem insignificant in another part of the body may prove to be intimately linked to oxidation and body malfunction.

To wrap up the antioxidants, I would like to specifically cover two of the most important ones—vitamin C and vitamin E, and how they offer protection to the body, but especially the brain. Why they are so important is that vitamin E protects fatty tissue because it is fat soluble, and vitamin C is water soluble so it protects the water part of the brain. In fact the brain is primarily made of made up of fat and water.

Vitamin C and vitamin E work together in the brain. Vitamin E neutralizers toxic oxidants and then vitamin C recycles the vitamin E residue and makes it active again. Vitamin E protects fatty acids in the brain, and by doing so, plays a crucial role in the early stages of memory loss and dementia.

We can now bring selenium—an antioxidant mineral into the equation. Vitamin E and selenium are closely linked and work together. One of their functions is to prevent viruses from altering genetic messages.

And it is also important to remember that metabolic enzymes play a key role in helping to protect the body. Without these enzymes the body would be unable to perform the billions of actions it generates each day to ensure that you are able to do all the different activities you are involved in, and also to ensure that you stay well and healthy.

It is therefore important to ensure that you eat a healthy diet to make sure that you get a plentiful supply of digestive enzymes to help the body perform its digestive function. This will ensure that your body has the necessary nutrients it requires to manufacture the many different metabolic enzymes it needs. If your diet is lacking in digestive enzymes, then you may like to consider topping up with a good, natural digestive enzyme supplement.

With regard to vitamin supplements, it is always best to take natural vitamin supplements as opposed to synthetic ones. Natural vitamin supplements have a life force within them, something that a synthetic one does not have. You often see very cheap vitamins advertised which are usually synthetic in origin.   You should ask yourself, would I rather put a chemical element in my body or a natural one? The natural form of vitamin E is called d-alpha tocopherol and the synthetic one dl-alpha tocopherol. There is not much difference in the name is there? And it is so easy to buy the wrong one.

So, along with your five servings each day of antioxidant rich fruit and vegetables, you may want to consider topping up with extra antioxidant supplements: vitamin E, C and beta carotene along with the minerals selenium and zinc. In addition, consider the herbs ginkgo biloba and turmeric as well.

Some good food sources of antioxidants include:

Allium sulphur compounds
Leeks, onions, and garlic.

Anthocyanins
Eggplant, grapes, and berries.

Beta-carotene
Pumpkin, mangoes, apricots, carrots, spinach, and parsley.

Catechins
Red wine and green tea.

Copper
Seafood, lean meat, milk, and nuts.

Cryptoxanthins
Red capsicum, pumpkin, and mangoes.

Flavonoids
Tea, green tea, citrus fruits, red wine, onion, and apples.

Indoles
Cruciferous vegetables such as broccoli, cabbage, and cauliflower.

Isoflavonoids
Soybeans, tofu, lentils, peas, and milk.

Lignans
Sesame seeds, bran, whole grains, and vegetables.

Lutein
Leafy greens like spinach and corn.

Lycopene
Tomatoes, pink grapefruit, and watermelon.

Manganese
Seafood, lean meat, milk, and nuts.

Polyphenols
Thyme and oregano.

Selenium
Seafood, offal, lean meat, and whole grains.

Vitamin C
Oranges, blackcurrants, kiwi fruit, mangoes, broccoli, spinach, capsicum, and strawberries.

Vitamin E
Vegetable oils (such as wheat germ oil), avocados, nuts, seeds, and whole grains.

Zinc
Seafood, lean meat, milk, and nuts.

Zoochemicals
Red meat, offal, and fish (Also derived from the plants that animals eat.)

To Sum Up

Many different things affect the production of amino acids and enzymes. The quality of the diet has a huge impact on the health of the body. If essential nutrients are lacking in the diet, then there could be a significant dietary shortfall of essential nutrients that the body needs to perform its billions of daily functions.

Another factor is what is often referred to as "if you eat a balanced diet then you will get all the nutrients your body needs." However, no one has yet been able to explain to me what a balanced diet is. Someone who has a very demanding physical job has very different nutritional requirements to someone who has a more sedentary occupation.

Likewise, someone who is involved in power sports has very different nutritional requirements than someone who is more advanced in years and is retired.

The quality of food today is nowhere as nutritious as it was say 50 years ago. Intensive farming practices using pesticides and fertilizers have robbed the land of much of its mineral content. Likewise, animal husbandry has seen dramatic changes in that the use of growth hormones and antibiotics is in widespread use today. And remember, all these hormone growth promoters and antibiotics can wind up in your body. Add this to lifestyle choices and any medication that may be taken for health conditions and the body has an uphill battle to fight in order to provide you with the energy that your lifestyle demands.

The purpose of this book has been to give you an insight into the fascinating subject of amino acids and enzymes. It is important to bear in mind that as a person ages their production of enzymes—especially in the pancreas declines significantly. Therefore many people make the decision to use enzyme and amino acids supplements to make up for this loss and also to counteract any dietary shortfall.

Many different products are available either from drugstores, supermarkets or on the Internet. There is a lot of hype surrounding enzyme and amino acid supplements—and some wild unsupported claims are made for some of them. You should remember the old adage—if the claim sounds too good to be true, then it probably is.

In order to get the maximum benefit for your money, you should only buy these types of supplements which are produced by a well know manufacturer, who has a good reputation to protect. And only buy natural products as opposed to synthetic ones. Natural supplements have a life force in them—they are living things, unlike synthetic ones which have no life force at all and are often by-products of the chemical industry. I know which one I would rather have in my body.

It is up to you how you provide your body with the nutrients it needs to support your lifestyle. Always listen to what your body is telling you. Make sure that you get adequate exercise, rest and sleep. Look after your body, Remember it is the only one that you have.

About The Author

Brian B Jacques has been a natural health researcher for over thirty years. He has presented seminars worldwide on such diverse subjects as Health Related issues, Motivation and Personal Development. In addition he has written numerous books, newsletters and articles on these subjects.

His very popular Series of Mini-Health Books includes:

- An Easy Way To Understand Eczema and Psoriasis
- An Easy Way To Understand Stress and Depression
- An Easy Way To Understand Parasites, Worms, Candida, Constipation and Detoxing
- An Easy Way To Understand Vitamins and Minerals
- An Easy Way To Understand Crohn's Disease and IBD
- An Easy Way To Understand Body Building For Men And Women
- An Easy Way To Understand Alzheimer's Disease
- An Easy Way To Understand Herpes
- An Easy Way To Understand Parkinson's Disease
- An Easy Way To Understand Autism
- An Easy Way To Understand Fibromyalgia
- The Little A–Z Dictionary of Herbal Remedies
- Effective Methods To Stop Smoking
- The Magic Of Vitamins & Minerals
- An Easy Way To Understand Your Body Systems
- An Easy Way To Understand Erectile Dysfunction
- An Easy Way To Understand Heart Disease, High Blood Pressure & Stroke
- An Easy Way To Understand Detoxing For Men & Women
- How To Lose Weight After 40
- How To Lose Weight And Maintain Your Ideal Weight Permanently
- Herbs For Healing - 101 Herbal Remedies

Another thirty titles in the Mini-Health Series are currently in preparation.

All these books are available as Kindle Editions (available from the Kindle Store on Amazon.com, and other countries Amazon sites where the Kindle platform is supported.) Many of these books are also available for the Barnes and Noble "Nook".

In addition, all these titles will shortly be available as print editions from the Amazon website.

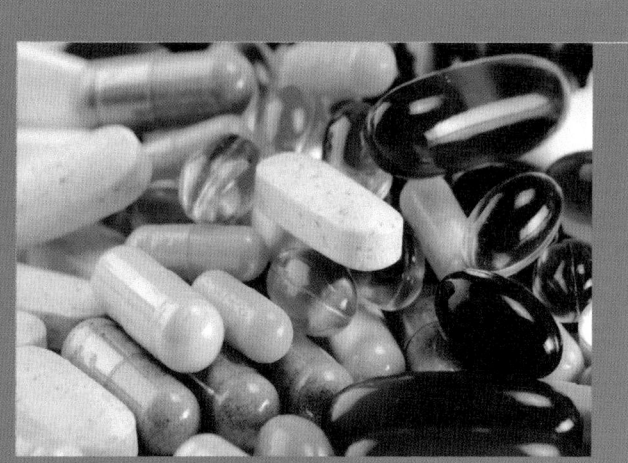

18333595R00026

Printed in Great Britain
by Amazon